How Genes Work

Table of Contents

What are proteins and what do they do?

Proteins are large, complex molecules that play many critical roles in the body. They do most of the work in cells and are required for the structure, function, and regulation of the body's tissues and organs.

Proteins are made up of hundreds or thousands of smaller units called amino acids, which are attached to one another in long chains. There are 20 different types of amino acids that can be combined to make a protein. The sequence of amino acids determines each protein's unique 3-dimensional structure and its specific function.

Proteins can be described according to their large range of functions in the body, listed in alphabetical order:

Examples of protein functions

Function	Description	Example
Antibody	Antibodies bind to specific foreign particles, such as viruses and bacteria, to help protect the body.	Immunoglobulin G (IgG) (image on page 4)
Enzyme	Enzymes carry out almost all of the thousands of chemical reactions that take place in cells. They also assist with the formation of new molecules by reading the genetic information stored in DNA.	Phenylalanine hydroxylase (image on page 5)
Messenger	Messenger proteins, such as some types of hormones, transmit signals to coordinate biological processes between different cells, tissues, and organs.	Growth hormone (image on page 6)
Structural component	These proteins provide structure and support for cells. On a larger scale, they also allow the body to move.	Actin (image on page 7)
Transport/ storage	These proteins bind and carry atoms and small molecules within cells and throughout the body.	Ferritin (image on page 8)

For more information about proteins and their functions:

KidsHealth from Nemours offers a basic overview of proteins (http://kidshealth.org/en/kids/protein.html) and what they do.

Arizona State University's "Ask a Biologist" discusses the different kinds of proteins (http://askabiologist.asu.edu/venom/what-are-proteins) and what they do.

Images

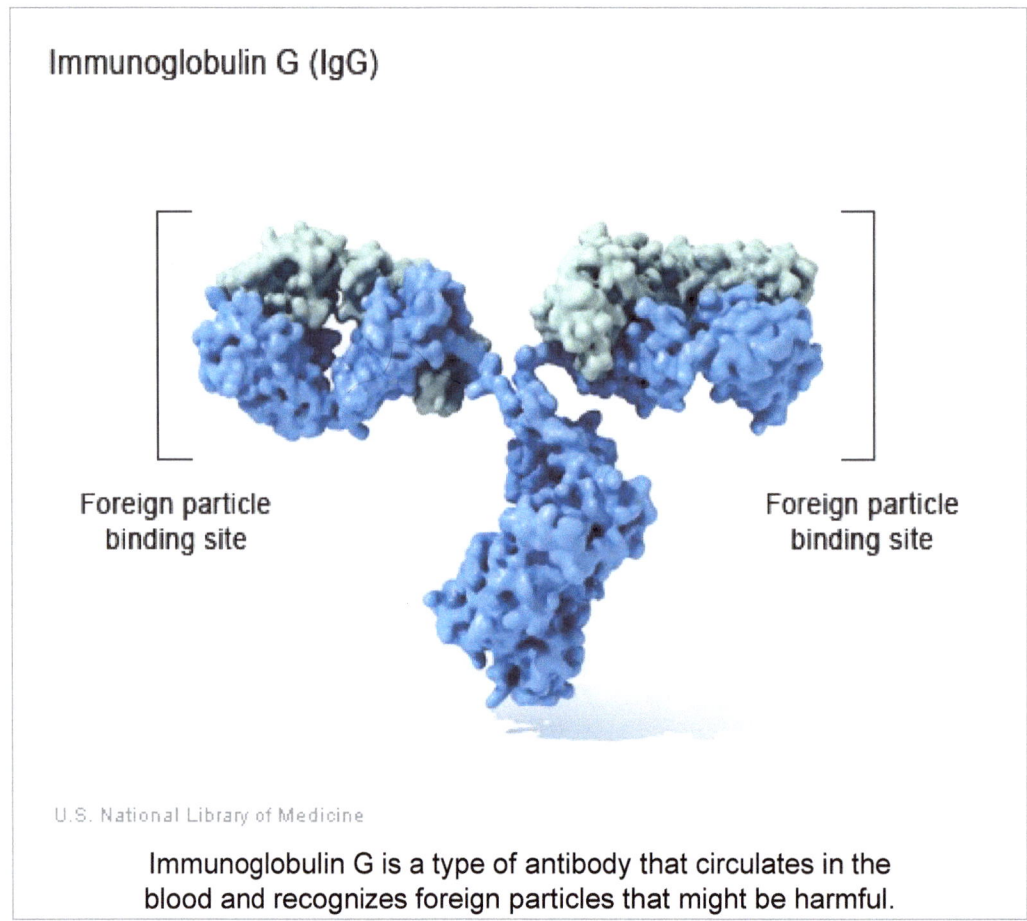

Immunoglobulin G (IgG)

Foreign particle
binding site

Foreign particle
binding site

U.S. National Library of Medicine

Immunoglobulin G is a type of antibody that circulates in the
blood and recognizes foreign particles that might be harmful.

Phenylalanine hydroxylase

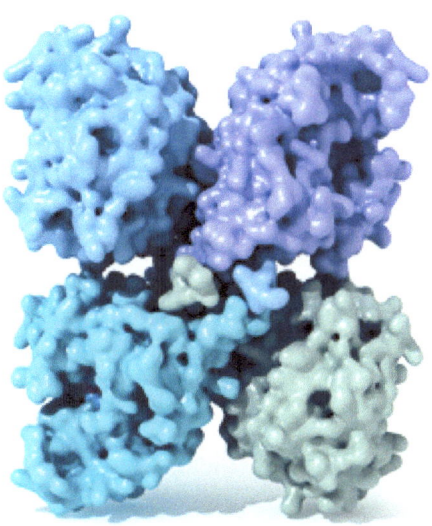

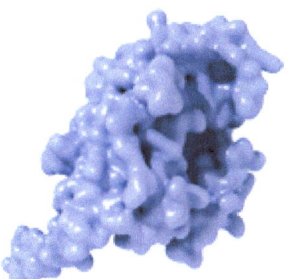

Single phenylalanine
hydroxylase subunit

Phenylalanine hydroxylase
protein consisting of 4 subunits

U.S. National Library of Medicine

The functional phenylalanine hydroxylase enzyme is made
up of four identical subunits. The enzyme converts the
amino acid phenylalanine to another amino acid, tyrosine.

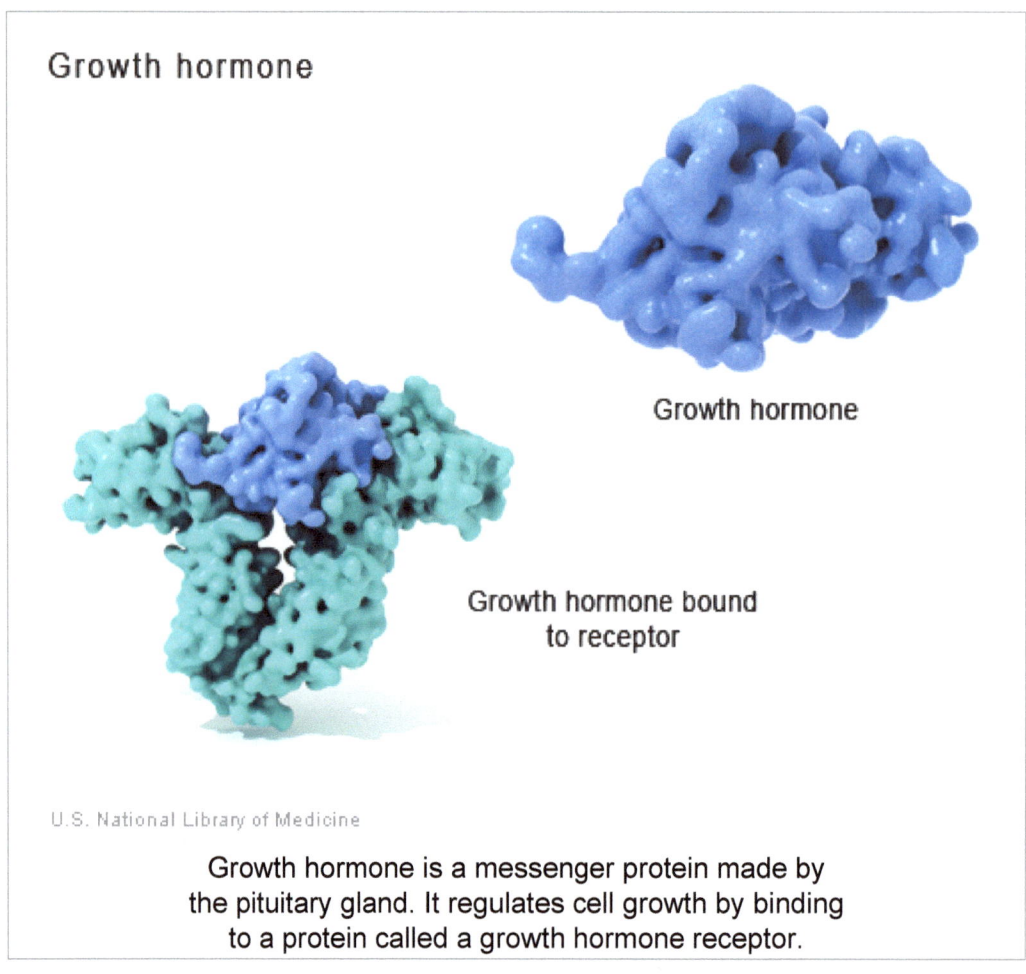

Growth hormone

Growth hormone

Growth hormone bound
to receptor

U.S. National Library of Medicine

Growth hormone is a messenger protein made by
the pituitary gland. It regulates cell growth by binding
to a protein called a growth hormone receptor.

Actin

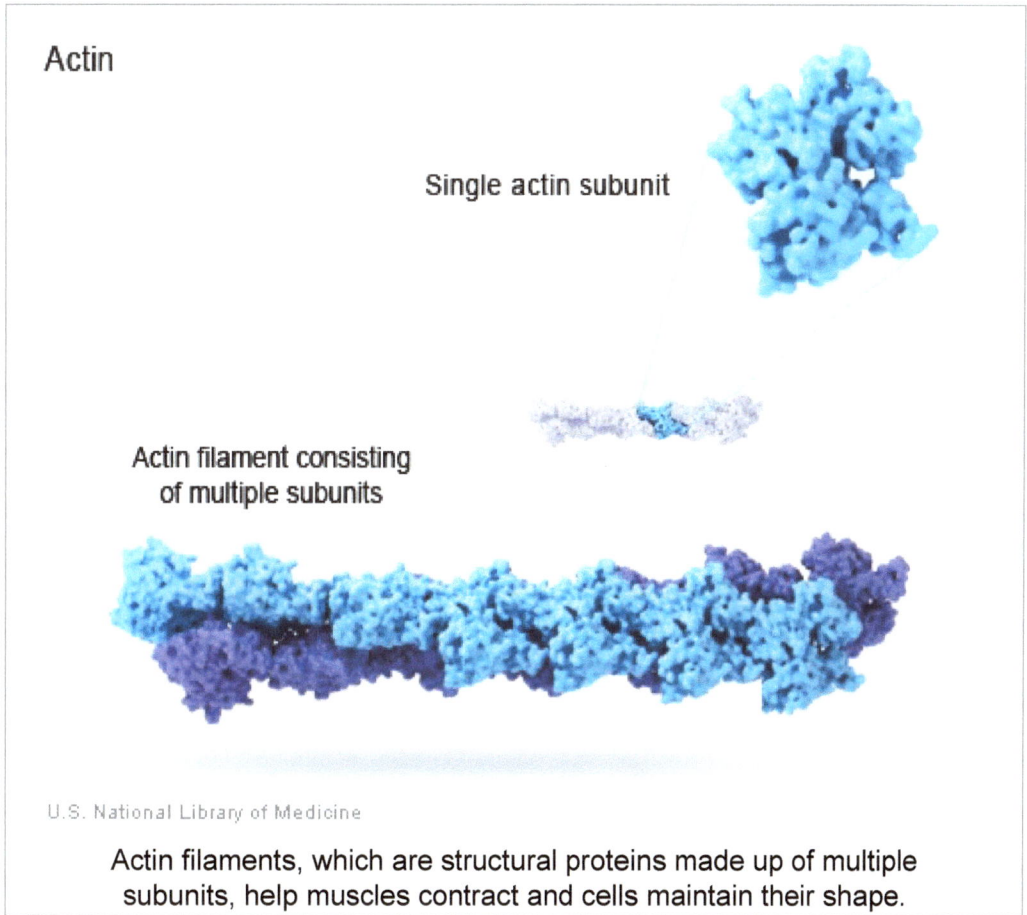

Single actin subunit

Actin filament consisting
of multiple subunits

U.S. National Library of Medicine

Actin filaments, which are structural proteins made up of multiple
subunits, help muscles contract and cells maintain their shape.

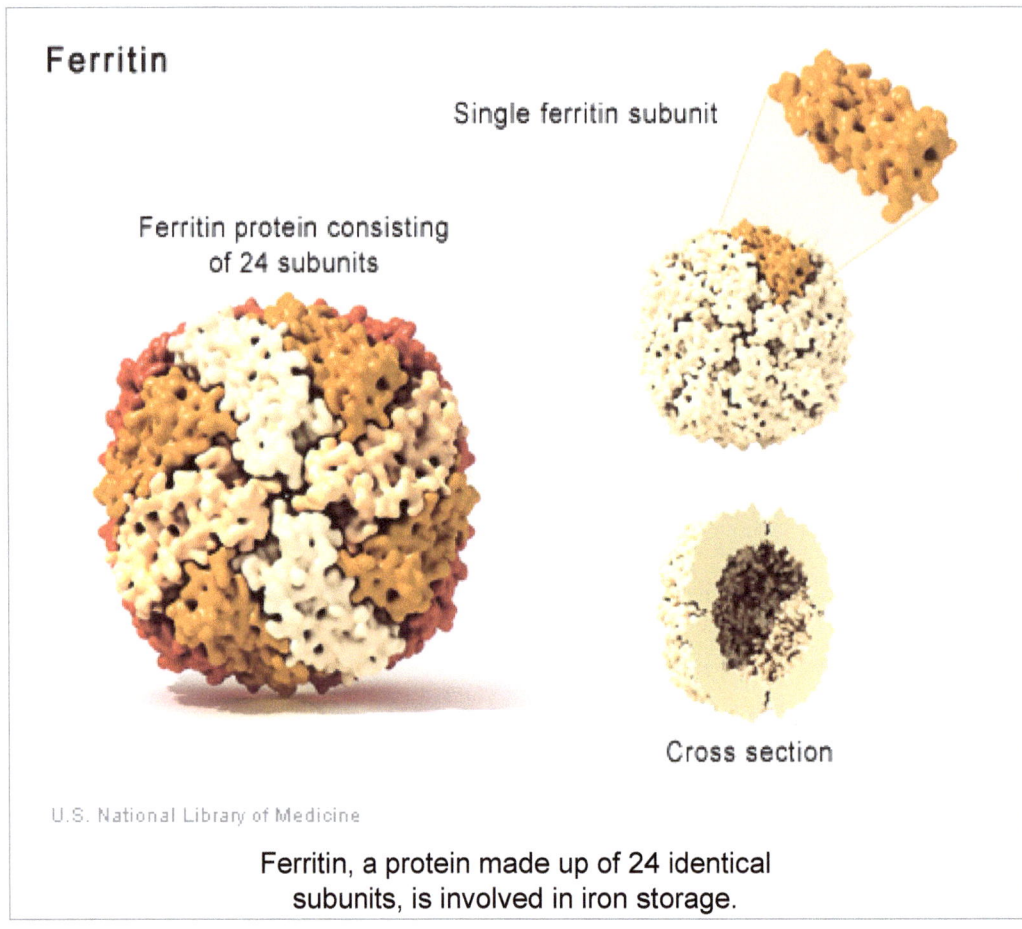

Ferritin

Single ferritin subunit

Ferritin protein consisting
of 24 subunits

Cross section

U.S. National Library of Medicine

Ferritin, a protein made up of 24 identical
subunits, is involved in iron storage.

How do genes direct the production of proteins?

Most genes contain the information needed to make functional molecules called proteins. (A few genes produce other molecules that help the cell assemble proteins.) The journey from gene to protein is complex and tightly controlled within each cell. It consists of two major steps: transcription and translation. Together, transcription and translation are known as gene expression.

During the process of transcription, the information stored in a gene's DNA is transferred to a similar molecule called RNA (ribonucleic acid) in the cell nucleus. Both RNA and DNA are made up of a chain of nucleotide bases, but they have slightly different chemical properties. The type of RNA that contains the information for making a protein is called messenger RNA (mRNA) because it carries the information, or message, from the DNA out of the nucleus into the cytoplasm.

Translation, the second step in getting from a gene to a protein, takes place in the cytoplasm. The mRNA interacts with a specialized complex called a ribosome, which "reads" the sequence of mRNA bases. Each sequence of three bases, called a codon, usually codes for one particular amino acid. (Amino acids are the building blocks of proteins.) A type of RNA called transfer RNA (tRNA) assembles the protein, one amino acid at a time. Protein assembly continues until the ribosome encounters a "stop" codon (a sequence of three bases that does not code for an amino acid).

The flow of information from DNA to RNA to proteins is one of the fundamental principles of molecular biology. It is so important that it is sometimes called the "central dogma."

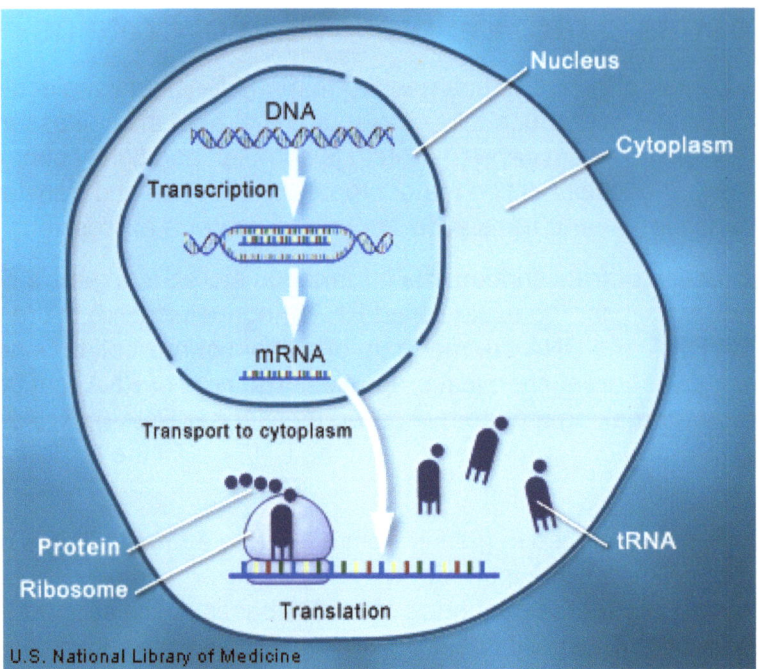

Through the processes of transcription and translation,
information from genes is used to make proteins.

For more information about making proteins:

The Genetic Science Learning Center at the University of Utah offers
an interactive introduction to transcription and translation (http://
learn.genetics.utah.edu/content/basics/dna).

Information about RNA (https://geneed.nlm.nih.gov/topic_subtopic.php?
tid=15&sid=18), transcription (https://geneed.nlm.nih.gov/topic_subtopic.php?
tid=15&sid=22), and translation (https://geneed.nlm.nih.gov/topic_subtopic.php?
tid=15&sid=23) is available from GeneEd.

North Dakota State University's Virtual Cell Animation Collection offers videos
that illustrate the processes of transcription (http://vcell.ndsu.nodak.edu/
animations/transcription/movie-flash.htm) and translation (http://
vcell.ndsu.nodak.edu/animations/translation/movie-flash.htm).

The New Genetics, a publication of the National Institute of General
Medical Sciences, includes discussions of transcription (https://
publications.nigms.nih.gov/thenewgenetics/chapter1.html#c4) and translation
(https://publications.nigms.nih.gov/thenewgenetics/chapter1.html#c7).

Can genes be turned on and off in cells?

Each cell expresses, or turns on, only a fraction of its genes. The rest of the genes are repressed, or turned off. The process of turning genes on and off is known as gene regulation. Gene regulation is an important part of normal development. Genes are turned on and off in different patterns during development to make a brain cell look and act different from a liver cell or a muscle cell, for example. Gene regulation also allows cells to react quickly to changes in their environments. Although we know that the regulation of genes is critical for life, this complex process is not yet fully understood.

Gene regulation can occur at any point during gene expression, but most commonly occurs at the level of transcription (when the information in a gene's DNA is transferred to mRNA). Signals from the environment or from other cells activate proteins called transcription factors. These proteins bind to regulatory regions of a gene and increase or decrease the level of transcription. By controlling the level of transcription, this process can determine the amount of protein product that is made by a gene at any given time.

For more information about gene regulation:

The Genetic Science Learning Center at the University of Utah offers an explanation of gene expression as it relates to disease risk (http://learn.genetics.utah.edu/content/science/expression/).

Additional information about gene expression (http://www.yourgenome.org/facts/what-is-gene-expression) is available from yourgenome.org, a service of the Wellcome Trust.

What is the epigenome?

DNA modifications that do not change the DNA sequence can affect gene activity. Chemical compounds that are added to single genes can regulate their activity; these modifications are known as epigenetic changes. The epigenome comprises all of the chemical compounds that have been added to the entirety of one's DNA (genome) as a way to regulate the activity (expression) of all the genes within the genome. The chemical compounds of the epigenome are not part of the DNA sequence, but are on or attached to DNA ("epi-" means above in Greek). Epigenomic modifications remain as cells divide and in some cases can be inherited through the generations. Environmental influences, such as a person's diet and exposure to pollutants, can also impact the epigenome.

Epigenetic changes can help determine whether genes are turned on or off and can influence the production of proteins in certain cells, ensuring that only necessary proteins are produced. For example, proteins that promote bone growth are not produced in muscle cells. Patterns of epigenome modification vary among individuals, different tissues within an individual, and even different cells.

A common type of epigenomic modification is called methylation. Methylation involves attaching small molecules called methyl groups, each consisting of one carbon atom and three hydrogen atoms, to segments of DNA. When methyl groups are added to a particular gene, that gene is turned off or silenced, and no protein is produced from that gene.

Because errors in the epigenetic process, such as modifying the wrong gene or failing to add a compound to a gene, can lead to abnormal gene activity or inactivity, they can cause genetic disorders. Conditions including cancers, metabolic disorders, and degenerative disorders have all been found to be related to epigenetic errors.

Scientists continue to explore the relationship between the genome and the chemical compounds that modify it. In particular, they are studying what effect the modifications have on gene function, protein production, and human health.

For more information about the epigenome:

The National Institutes of Health (NIH) offers the NIH Roadmap Epigenomics Project (http://www.roadmapepigenomics.org/), which provides epigenome maps of a variety of cells to begin to assess the relationship between epigenomics and human disease.

The National Center for Biotechnology Information (NCBI) provides the NCBI Epigenomics (http://www.ncbi.nlm.nih.gov/epigenomics) database of maps of the epigenomes of various species and many cell types.

Human Epigenome Atlas (http://www.genboree.org/epigenomeatlas/index.rhtml) from Baylor College of Medicine allows for comparison of the epigenomes of many species and cell types.

GeneEd from the National Library of Medicine and the National Human Genome Research Institute provides a list of educational resources about the epigenome (https://geneed.nlm.nih.gov/topic_subtopic.php?tid=35&sid=36).

Ongoing research is being done with the Human Epigenome Project (http://www.epigenome.org/).

The University of Utah provides an interactive epigenetics tutorial (http://learn.genetics.utah.edu/content/epigenetics/).

The National Human Genome Research Institute provides a fact sheet (https://www.genome.gov/27532724) on Epigenomics.

Many tools for understanding epigenomics are available through the NIH Common Fund Epigenomics Project (https://commonfund.nih.gov/epigenomics/).

How do cells divide?

There are two types of cell division: mitosis and meiosis. Most of the time when people refer to "cell division," they mean mitosis, the process of making new body cells. Meiosis is the type of cell division that creates egg and sperm cells.

Mitosis is a fundamental process for life. During mitosis, a cell duplicates all of its contents, including its chromosomes, and splits to form two identical daughter cells. Because this process is so critical, the steps of mitosis are carefully controlled by a number of genes. When mitosis is not regulated correctly, health problems such as cancer can result.

The other type of cell division, meiosis, ensures that humans have the same number of chromosomes in each generation. It is a two-step process that reduces the chromosome number by half—from 46 to 23—to form sperm and egg cells. When the sperm and egg cells unite at conception, each contributes 23 chromosomes so the resulting embryo will have the usual 46. Meiosis also allows genetic variation through a process of DNA shuffling while the cells are dividing.

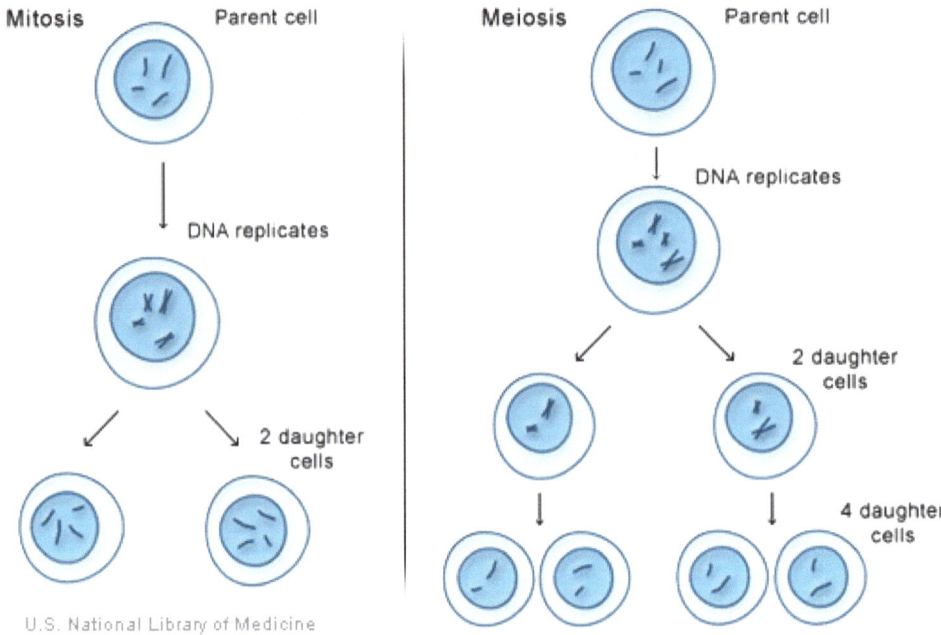

Mitosis and meiosis, the two types of cell division.

For more information about cell division:

Information about mitosis (https://geneed.nlm.nih.gov/topic_subtopic.php?
tid=1&sid=2) and meiosis (https://geneed.nlm.nih.gov/topic_subtopic.php?
tid=1&sid=3) is available from GeneEd.

North Dakota State University's Virtual Cell Animation Collection offers videos
that illustrate the processes of mitosis (http://vcell.ndsu.nodak.edu/animations/
mitosis/movie-flash.htm) and meiosis (http://vcell.ndsu.nodak.edu/animations/
meiosis/movie-flash.htm).

Yourgenome from the Wellcome Trust outlines the similarities and differences
between mitosis and meiosis (http://www.yourgenome.org/facts/mitosis-versus-
meiosis).

How do genes control the growth and division of cells?

A variety of genes are involved in the control of cell growth and division. The cell cycle is the cell's way of replicating itself in an organized, step-by-step fashion. Tight regulation of this process ensures that a dividing cell's DNA is copied properly, any errors in the DNA are repaired, and each daughter cell receives a full set of chromosomes. The cycle has checkpoints (also called restriction points), which allow certain genes to check for mistakes and halt the cycle for repairs if something goes wrong.

If a cell has an error in its DNA that cannot be repaired, it may undergo programmed cell death (apoptosis) (image on page 17). Apoptosis is a common process throughout life that helps the body get rid of cells it doesn't need. Cells that undergo apoptosis break apart and are recycled by a type of white blood cell called a macrophage (image on page 17). Apoptosis protects the body by removing genetically damaged cells that could lead to cancer, and it plays an important role in the development of the embryo and the maintenance of adult tissues.

Cancer results from a disruption of the normal regulation of the cell cycle. When the cycle proceeds without control, cells can divide without order and accumulate genetic defects that can lead to a cancerous tumor (image on page 18).

For more information about cell growth and division:

The National Institutes of Health's Apoptosis Interest Group (http://sigs.nih.gov/cell-death/Pages/Miscellaneous.aspx) provides an introduction to programmed cell death.

The National Cancer Institute's fact sheet What is Cancer? (http://www.cancer.gov/about-cancer/what-is-cancer) explains the growth of cancerous tumors.

Images

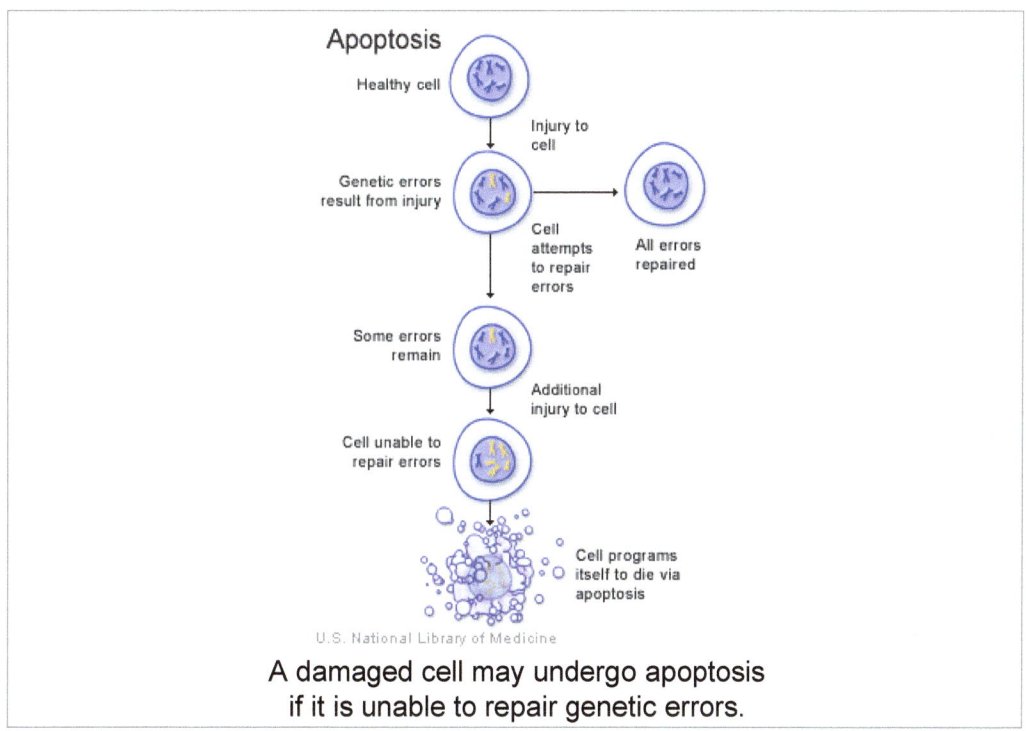

A damaged cell may undergo apoptosis
if it is unable to repair genetic errors.

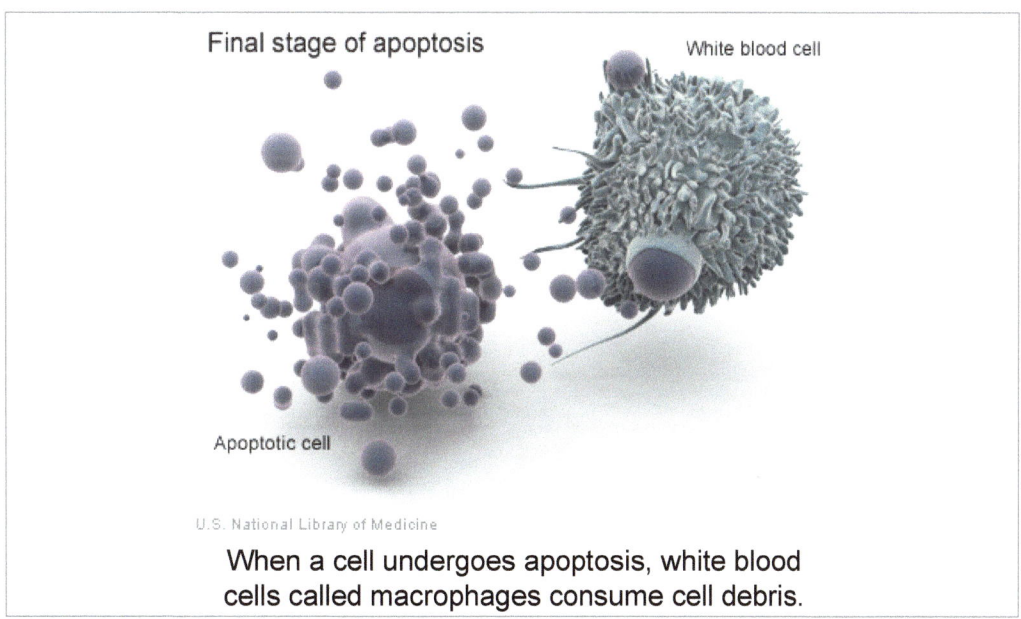

When a cell undergoes apoptosis, white blood
cells called macrophages consume cell debris.

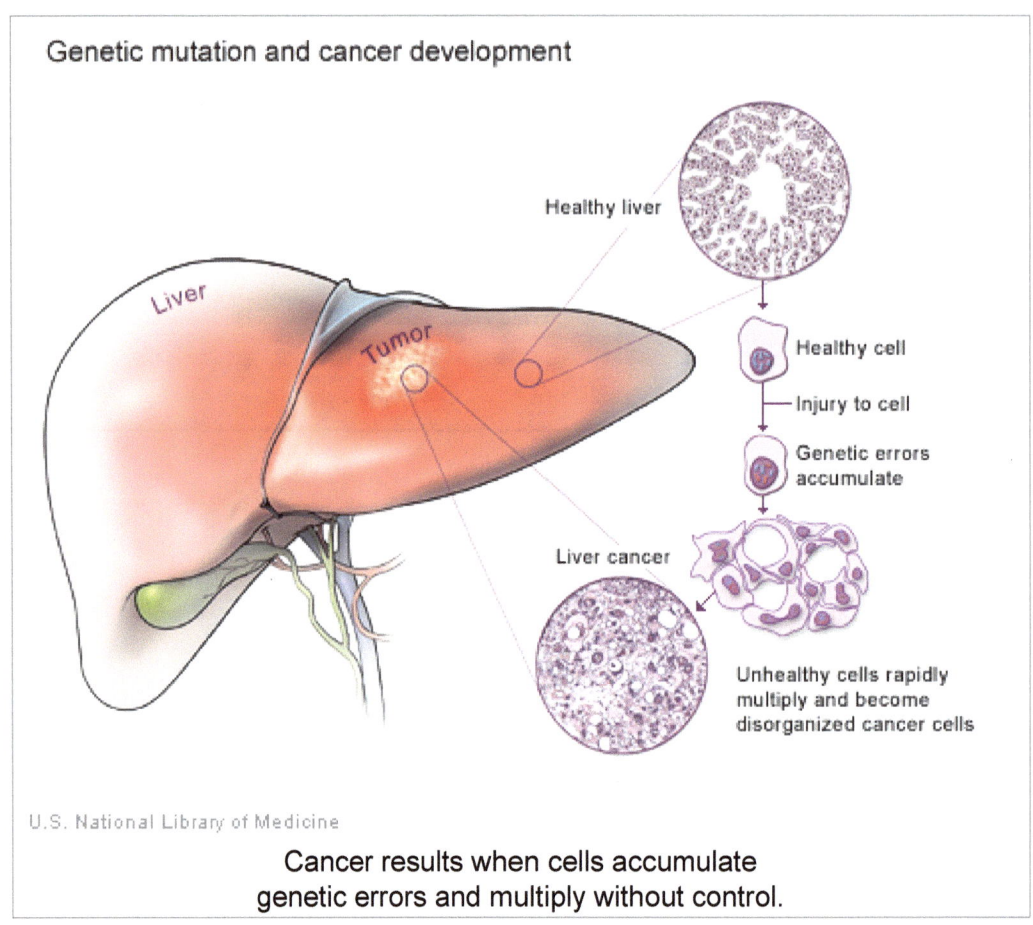

Genetic mutation and cancer development

Healthy liver

Liver

Tumor

Healthy cell

Injury to cell

Genetic errors
accumulate

Liver cancer

Unhealthy cells rapidly
multiply and become
disorganized cancer cells

U.S. National Library of Medicine

Cancer results when cells accumulate
genetic errors and multiply without control.

How do geneticists indicate the location of a gene?

Geneticists use maps to describe the location of a particular gene on a chromosome. One type of map uses the cytogenetic location to describe a gene's position. The cytogenetic location is based on a distinctive pattern of bands created when chromosomes are stained with certain chemicals. Another type of map uses the molecular location, a precise description of a gene's position on a chromosome. The molecular location is based on the sequence of DNA building blocks (base pairs) that make up the chromosome.

Cytogenetic location

Geneticists use a standardized way of describing a gene's cytogenetic location. In most cases, the location describes the position of a particular band on a stained chromosome:

17q12

It can also be written as a range of bands, if less is known about the exact location:

17q12-q21

The combination of numbers and letters provide a gene's "address" on a chromosome. This address is made up of several parts:

- The chromosome on which the gene can be found. The first number or letter used to describe a gene's location represents the chromosome. Chromosomes 1 through 22 (the autosomes) are designated by their chromosome number. The sex chromosomes are designated by X or Y.
- The arm of the chromosome. Each chromosome is divided into two sections (arms) based on the location of a narrowing (constriction) called the centromere. By convention, the shorter arm is called p, and the longer arm is called q. The chromosome arm is the second part of the gene's address. For example, 5q is the long arm of chromosome 5, and Xp is the short arm of the X chromosome.

- The position of the gene on the p or q arm. The position of a gene is based on a distinctive pattern of light and dark bands that appear when the chromosome is stained in a certain way. The position is usually designated by two digits (representing a region and a band), which are sometimes followed by a decimal point and one or more additional digits (representing sub-bands within a light or dark area). The number indicating the gene position increases with distance from the centromere. For example: 14q21 represents position 21 on the long arm of chromosome 14. 14q21 is closer to the centromere than 14q22.

Sometimes, the abbreviations "cen" or "ter" are also used to describe a gene's cytogenetic location. "Cen" indicates that the gene is very close to the centromere. For example, 16pcen refers to the short arm of chromosome 16 near the centromere. "Ter" stands for terminus, which indicates that the gene is very close to the end of the p or q arm. For example, 14qter refers to the tip of the long arm of chromosome 14. ("Tel" is also sometimes used to describe a gene's location. "Tel" stands for telomeres, which are at the ends of each chromosome. The abbreviations "tel" and "ter" refer to the same location.)

Chromosomal location of a gene

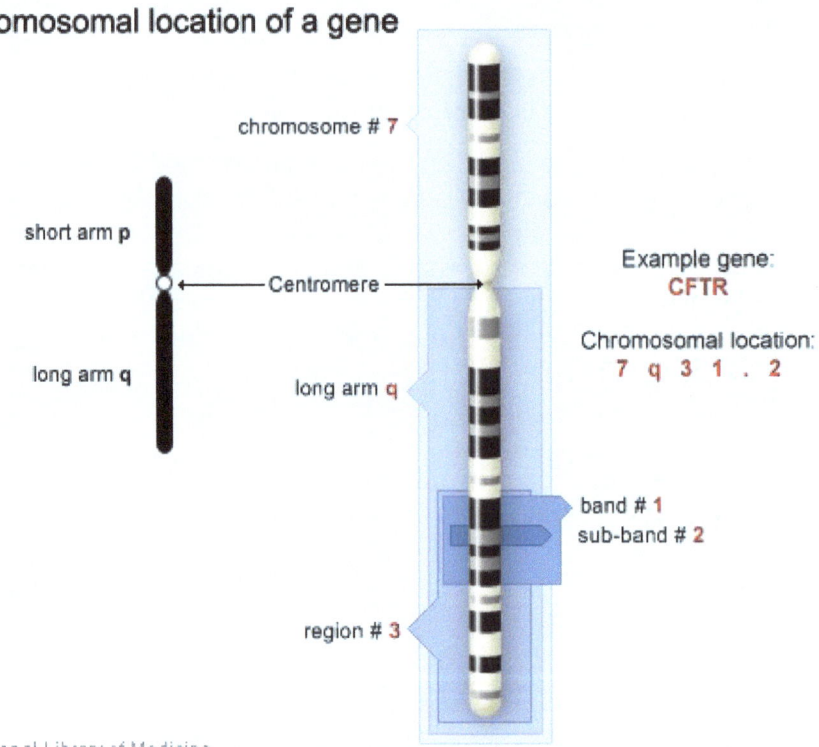

The CFTR gene is located on the long arm of chromosome 7 at position 7q31.2.

Molecular location

The Human Genome Project, an international research effort completed in 2003, determined the sequence of base pairs for each human chromosome. This sequence information allows researchers to provide a more specific address than the cytogenetic location for many genes. A gene's molecular address pinpoints the location of that gene in terms of base pairs. It describes the gene's precise position on a chromosome and indicates the size of the gene. Knowing the molecular location also allows researchers to determine exactly how far a gene is from other genes on the same chromosome.

Different groups of researchers often present slightly different values for a gene's molecular location. Researchers interpret the sequence of the human genome using a variety of methods, which can result in small differences in a gene's molecular address. Genetics Home Reference presents data from NCBI (http://www.ncbi.nlm.nih.gov/sites/entrez?db=gene) for the molecular location of genes.

For more information on genetic mapping:

The National Human Genome Research Institute explains how researchers create a genetic map (https://www.genome.gov/10000715).

The University of Washington provides a Cytogenetics Gallery (http://www.pathology.washington.edu/galleries/Cytogallery/main.php?file=intro) that includes a description of chromosome banding patterns (http://www.pathology.washington.edu/galleries/Cytogallery/main.php?file=banding+patterns).

Information about assembling and annotating the genome (http://www.ncbi.nlm.nih.gov/bookshelf/br.fcgi?book=handbook&part=ch14) is available from NCBI.

www.ingramcontent.com/pod-product-compliance
Lightning Source LLC
Chambersburg PA
CBHW050913180526

45159CB00007B/2902